GUIDELINES TO NATURALLY LOSS OVERWEIGHT
Learn The Tested Ways On How You Can Loss Weight Naturally

EMMANUEL YERMAKOV

Table of contents

Chapter 1

Chapter 2

Chapter 3

Chapter 4

Chapter 1

Obesity is typically described as having too much bodily mass. A BMI of 30 or greater is the accepted criterion for obesity in adults. A BMI of 40 or greater is considered extreme obesity. Childhood obesity is assessed against growth charts.
Obesity may create health concerns throughout your body.
Obesity has direct and indirect impacts on various physiological systems.

What is obesity?
Obesity is a complicated, chronic condition with various factors that contribute to excessive body fat and occasionally, poor health. Body fat itself is not an illness, of course. But when your body

has too much additional fat, it might affect the way it operates. These alterations are gradual, may worsen over time, and they can lead to significant health outcomes.

The good news is that you can improve your health risks by shedding part of your extra body fat. Even tiny changes in weight may have a major influence on your health. Not every weight reduction approach works for everyone. Most individuals have attempted to reduce weight more than once. And keeping the weight off is just as crucial as losing it in the first place.

Worldwide, obesity has roughly quadrupled in the previous 50 years. The surge has been particularly striking in lower-income nations where malnutrition is endemic. These populations now have increased access to higher-calorie items with less nutritional value. Obesity now regularly coexists with undernutrition in these nations.

Chapter 2

What causes obesity and overweight in our body?

On the most basic level, obesity is caused by ingesting more calories than your body can utilize. Many variables contribute to this. Some elements are particular to you. Others are built into the framework of our society, either on a national, local, or familial level. In some respects, avoiding obesity entails intentionally acting against these numerous causes.

Screen culture. As work, shopping and social life continue to shift online, we progressively spend more time in front of our phones and computers. Streaming media and binge-watching make long hours of inactive enjoyment more feasible.

Workforce changes. With industrial trends going toward automation and technology, more individuals today work at desks than on their feet. They also work longer hours.

Fatigue. Sedentary lifestyles have a snowball effect. Studies demonstrate that the longer you remain motionless, the wearier and less motivated you become. Sitting makes your body rigid and adds to aches and pains that hinder activity. It also produces overall tension, which contributes to weariness.

Neighborhood design. Many individuals lack local venues to be active, either due to access or safety reasons. More than half of Americans don't live within half a mile of a park. They may not live in walkable areas, and they may not see others in their communities being active in day-to-day living. When there is no public transit alternative, most individuals can only commute by automobile.

Childcare trends. Children spend less time playing outdoors than they used to. They spend more time in confined daycare spaces, which may not offer appropriate rooms or facilities for physical exercise. This is partially due to societal tendencies that don't think it safe for youngsters to play outdoors unsupervised. It's also related to poor access to public areas and inadequate availability of decent daycare. Many daycare facilities replace TV for free play.

Disability. Adults and children with physical and learning challenges are particularly at risk for obesity. Physical restrictions and lack of proper specialist knowledge and resources might contribute.

More importantly, when you come to your healthcare provider for treatment, they will want to know your full health narrative. They will question you about your history of medical issues, medicines, and weight fluctuations. They'll also want to hear about your current eating, sleeping, and activity practices and stress factors and if you have attempted any weight reduction programs in the past. They may question your biological family's health history.

They will also assess your vital functions by measuring your heart rate and blood pressure and listening to your heart and lungs. They may offer you a blood test to assess your blood glucose and cholesterol levels and screen for hormone abnormalities. They'll utilize this comprehensive profile to identify your obesity and any linked illnesses you could have.

The dietary modifications you individually need to make to lose weight will be particular to you. Some individuals may benefit from lowering portion amounts or snacking between meals. For others, it may be more about modifying what they eat than how much. Almost everyone can benefit from eating more vegetables. Fruits, vegetables, whole grains, and legumes tend to be lower in fat and richer in fiber and minerals. They are more nutritious and might help you feel fuller and more pleased after eating fewer calories.

Increased activity
Everyone has heard that food and exercise are both vital to weight reduction and weight

maintenance. But exercising doesn't have to require a gym membership.

Just walking at a moderate speed is one of the most effective methods of exercise for weight reduction. Just 30 minutes, five days a week is what healthcare professionals urge. A regular stroll at lunchtime or before or after work may make a huge impact.

Make a tiny sacrifice. Do you have a daily snack habit or "pick-me-up," such as a sweet drink, that is high in calories? Consider replacing it. Just 150 more calories a day might build up to 10 extra pounds in a year. That's comparable to a snack-size bag of potato chips, or only two double-stuffed Oreos.

Add a simple activity. Alternatively, think about what you would do to spend an additional 150 calories in a day. For example, go for a hike or use an elliptical machine for 25 minutes, or take the dog for a brisk walk for 35 minutes.

Shop deliberately. Stock your house with healthful meals and keep sweets and snacks for special occasions when you go out.

Whole foods are richer in fiber and lower on the glycemic index, so they don't cause your blood sugar to surge and plummet the way processed snacks and desserts do.

Cultivate overall well-being. Reduce your screen time, get outdoors and go for a stroll. Manage your stress and try to get appropriate sleep to keep your hormone levels in line. Focus on good improvements and healthy activities rather than how your efforts affect your weight.

Remember, weight reduction of merely 5% to 10% may considerably reduce your health risks. It may reduce or halt the development of fatty liver disease, metabolic syndrome, and diabetes. With medical direction, weight reduction of at least this amount is attainable, and maybe considerably more. Sticking with a long-term treatment plan will help you sustain weight reduction.

The good news is that as research progresses, advances in medicine continue to give fresh hope for managing obesity. It could take some investigating to arrive at the correct formula for you, but along with your healthcare practitioner, you can take your health back into your own hands. Even a little weight reduction may enhance your health on practically every level, and you can get lasting advantages from smart food and lifestyle adjustments.

Chapter 3

How can Overweight and obesity affect our body

How does fat influence my body?
Obesity impacts your body in various ways. Some are just the mechanical implications of having extra body fat. For example, you can draw a clear connection between increased weight on your body and greater strain on your bones and joints. Other impacts are more subtle, such as chemical changes in your blood that raise your risk for diabetes, heart disease, and stroke.

Some impacts are still not completely understood. For example, there is an increased risk of some malignancies with obesity. We don't know why, yet it exists. Statistically, obesity raises the chance of early mortality from all causes. By the same token, studies suggest that you may dramatically reduce these risks by dropping even a minor amount of weight (5% to 10%).

Metabolic alterations
Your metabolism is the process of turning food into energy to power your body's operations.

When your body has more calories than it can need, it turns the additional calories into lipids and stores them in your adipose tissue (body fat) (body fat). When you run out of tissue to store lipids in, the fat cells themselves get larger. Enlarged fat cells emit hormones and other substances that induce an inflammatory reaction.

Type 2 diabetes. Obesity especially elevates the risk of Type 2 diabetes seven-fold in persons assigned male at birth and 12-fold in those assigned female at birth. The risk rises by 20% for every extra point you acquire on the BMI scale. It also reduces weight reduction. Cardiovascular illnesses.

High blood pressure, excessive cholesterol, high blood sugar, and inflammation are all risk factors for cardiovascular disorders, including coronary artery disease, congestive heart failure, heart attack, and stroke. These hazards rise hand-in-hand with your BMI.

Cardiovascular disease is the biggest cause of avoidable mortality globally and in the U.S.

Fatty liver disease. Excess fats flowing in your blood find their way to your liver, which is responsible for purifying your blood. When your liver starts accumulating extra fat, it may lead to chronic liver inflammation (hepatitis) and long-term liver damage (cirrhosis) (cirrhosis).

extra body fat may cause Kidney disease. High blood pressure, diabetes, and liver disease are among the most prevalent factors of chronic kidney disease.

Excess body fat may overload the organs of your respiratory system and cause stress and pressure on your musculoskeletal system.

Chapter 4

Guidelines to lose weight naturally

28 Easy Ways to Lose Weight Naturally (Backed by Science) (Backed by Science)
There is a lot of bad weight loss material on the internet.

Much of what is advocated is dubious at best, and not based on any solid science.

However, some natural techniques have been demonstrated to work.

Here are 29 simple strategies to reduce weight naturally.

1. Add Protein to Your Diet
When it comes to weight reduction, protein is the king of nutrition.

Your body burns calories while digesting and metabolizing the protein you consume, therefore a high-protein diet may enhance metabolism by up to 80–100 calories per day.

A high-protein diet may also help you feel more full and lower your appetite. Several studies demonstrate that individuals consume nearly 400 fewer calories per day on a high-protein diet.

Even something as basic as having a high-protein meal (like eggs) may have a profound impact

2. Eat Whole, Single-Ingredient Foods
One of the finest things you can do to get healthy is to base your diet on whole, single-ingredient meals.

By doing this, you remove the great bulk of added sugar, added fat, and processed food.

Most whole meals are inherently quite full, making it a lot simpler to maintain safe calorie limits.

Furthermore, eating complete meals also offers your body the many critical nutrients that it needs to operate effectively.

Weight reduction typically comes as a natural side effect of consuming complete foods.

3. Avoid Processed Foods

Processed foods are frequently heavy in added sugars, extra fats, and calories.

What's more, processed meals are tailored to help you consume as much as possible. They are far more prone to create addictive-like eating than unprocessed meals.

4. Stock Up on Healthy Foods and Snacks

Studies have shown that the food you keep at home considerably influences weight and eating habits.

By constantly keeping nutritious food accessible, you limit the possibility of you or other family members eating unhealthy.

There are also numerous nutritious and natural snacks that are simple to make and carry with you on the road.

These include yogurt, whole fruit, almonds, carrots, and hard-boiled eggs.

5. Limit Your Intake of Added Sugar

Eating a lot of added sugar is related to several of the world's major illnesses, including heart disease, type 2 diabetes, and cancer.

On average, Americans consume around 15 teaspoons of added sugar per day. This quantity is generally buried in many processed meals, so you may be ingesting a lot of sugar without even realizing it.

Since sugar goes by many names in ingredient lists, it may be quite difficult to find out how much sugar a product truly contains.

Minimizing your consumption of added sugar is an excellent strategy to enhance your diet.

6. Drink Water

There is real validity to the idea that drinking water might aid with weight reduction.

Drinking 0.5 liters (17 oz) of water may boost the calories you burn by 24–30% for an hour thereafter.

Drinking water before meals may also contribute to lower calorie consumption, particularly for middle-aged and older persons.

Water is especially effective for weight reduction when it substitutes other drinks that are heavy in calories and sugar.

7. Drink (Unsweetened) Coffee

Fortunately, people are understanding that coffee is a healthful beverage that is filled with antioxidants and other helpful chemicals.

Coffee consumption may promote weight reduction by improving energy levels and the number of calories you burn.

Caffeinated coffee may boost your metabolism by 3–11% and reduce your risk of developing type 2 diabetes by a whopping 23–50%.

Furthermore, black coffee is particularly weight loss friendly, as it may make you feel full yet contains nearly no calories.

8. Limit the way you consume Liquid Calories

Liquid calories originate from beverages including sugary soft drinks, fruit juices, chocolate milk, and energy drinks.

These beverages are detrimental to health in various ways, including an increased risk of obesity. One research demonstrated a significant 60% increase in the incidence of obesity among youngsters, for each daily consumption of a sugar-sweetened beverage.

It's also crucial to remember that your brain does not register liquid calories the same way it does solid calories, so you end up putting these calories on top of everything else that you consume.

9. Limit Your Intake of Refined Carbs
Refined carbohydrates are carbs that have had most of their essential elements and fiber removed.

The refining procedure leaves nothing but readily absorbed carbohydrates, which might raise the risk of overeating and illness.

The primary dietary sources of refined carbohydrates include white flour, white bread, white rice, sodas, pastries, snacks, sweets, pasta, morning cereals, and added sugar.

10. Fast Intermittently

Intermittent fasting is an eating habit that alternates between periods of fasting and eating.

There are several various methods to conduct intermittent fasting, including the 5:2 diet, the 16:8 approach, and the eat-stop-eat strategy.

Generally, these approaches help you consume fewer calories overall, without having to intentionally control calories throughout the meal hours. This should contribute to weight reduction, as well as various other health advantages.

11. Drink (Unsweetened) Green Tea
Green tea is a natural beverage that is filled with antioxidants.

Drinking green tea is related to several advantages, such as enhanced fat burning and weight reduction.

Green tea may boost energy expenditure by 4% and enhance selective fat burning by up to 17%, particularly detrimental to belly fat.
Matcha green tea is a form of powdered green tea that may offer even more potent health benefits than normal green tea.

12. Eat More Fruits and Vegetables
Fruits and vegetables are incredibly nutritious, weight-loss-friendly foods.

In addition to being abundant in water, minerals, and fiber, they generally have relatively low energy density. This makes it feasible to consume huge amounts without absorbing too many calories.

Numerous studies have indicated that those who consume more fruits and vegetables tend to weigh less.

13. Count Calories Once in a While
Being conscious of what you're eating is incredibly beneficial while attempting to reduce weight.

There are various efficient methods to accomplish this, like tracking calories, maintaining a food journal, or taking photographs of what you eat.

Using an app or another electronic tool may be even more effective than writing in a food journal.

14. Use Smaller Plates

Some studies have indicated that using smaller plates helps you eat less since it affects how you view portion sizes.

People appear to load their plates the same, regardless of plate size, therefore they end up placing more food on bigger plates than on smaller ones.

Using smaller dishes minimizes how much food you consume while giving you the feeling of having eaten more.

15. Try a Low-Carb Diet

Many studies have demonstrated that low-carb diets are particularly helpful for weight reduction.

Limiting carbohydrates and eating more fat and protein lessens your appetite and helps you consume fewer calories.

This may result in weight reduction that is up to 3 times more than that with a conventional low-fat diet.

A low-carb diet may also lower numerous risk factors for illness.

16. Eat More Slowly

If you eat too rapidly, you may take significantly too many calories before your body even knows that you are full.

Faster eaters are far more prone to acquire obese, compared to individuals who eat more slowly.

Chewing more slowly may help you consume fewer calories and enhance the synthesis of hormones that are connected to weight reduction.

17. Add Eggs to Your Diet

Eggs are the best weight loss meal. They are inexpensive, low in calories, rich in protein, and filled with all kinds of nutrients.

High-protein meals have been demonstrated to lower hunger and promote fullness, compared to diets that contain less protein.

Furthermore, eating eggs for breakfast may induce up to 65% higher weight reduction over 8 weeks, compared to eating bagels for breakfast. It may also help you consume fewer calories during the remainder of the day.

18. Spice Up Your Meals

Chili peppers and jalapenos contain a chemical called capsaicin, which may improve metabolism and promote the burning of fat Capsaicin may also lower appetite and calorie consumption.

19. Get Enough Sleep
Getting adequate sleep is highly crucial for weight reduction, as well as to avoid future weight gain.

Studies have indicated that sleep-deprived adults are up to 55% more likely to acquire obese, compared to those who receive adequate sleep. This number is significantly greater for youngsters.

This is mainly because sleep deprivation alters the daily oscillations in appetite hormones, leading to poor appetite control.

20. Eat More Fiber ,Fiber-rich meals may aid with weight reduction.

Foods that include water-soluble fiber may be particularly useful, as this kind of fiber may aid boost the sense of fullness.

Fiber may delay stomach emptying, make the stomach enlarge, and enhance the production of satiety hormones.

Ultimately, this helps us eat less naturally, without having to think about it.

Furthermore, several forms of fiber help nourish the friendly gut flora. Healthy gut flora has been connected with a lower risk of obesity.

Just be careful to increase your fiber consumption gradually to minimize stomach discomfort, such as bloating, cramps, and diarrhea.

21. Brush Your Teeth After Meals
Many individuals clean or floss their teeth after eating, which may help minimize the temptation to snack or eat between meals.

This is because many individuals do not feel like eating after cleaning their teeth. Plus, it may make meals taste unpleasant.

Therefore, if you brush or use mouthwash after eating, you may be less motivated to grab an unneeded snack.

22. Combat Your Food Addiction
Food addiction includes intense cravings and changes in your brain chemistry that make it tougher to avoid eating particular foods.

This is a primary cause of overeating for many individuals and affects a considerable proportion of the population. A recent 2014 research indicated that approximately 20% of respondents fit the criteria for food addiction.

Some meals are far more prone to trigger signs of addiction than others. This includes highly processed junk foods that are heavy in sugar, fat, or both.

The greatest method to fight food addiction is to get treatment.

23. Do Some Sort of Cardio
Doing exercise — whether it is jogging, running, cycling, power walking, or hiking — is a terrific method to burn calories and enhance both mental and physical health.

Cardio has been demonstrated to improve numerous risk factors for heart disease. It may also help decrease body weight.
Cardio appears to be especially efficient in reducing the harmful belly fat that builds up around your organs and promotes metabolic illness.

24. Add Resistance Exercises
Loss of muscle mass is a typical adverse effect of dieting.

If you lose a lot of muscle, your body will start burning fewer calories than previously
By lifting weights consistently, you'll be able to avoid this decrease in muscle mass.
As an extra advantage, you'll also look and feel much better

25. Practice Mindful Eating
Mindful eating is a practice used to improve awareness when eating.

It helps you make thoughtful eating choices and increase awareness of your hunger and satiety indicators. It then helps you eat properly in response to those suggestions.
Mindful eating has been demonstrated to have substantial impacts on weight, eating behavior, and stress in patients with obesity. It is particularly beneficial against binge eating and emotional eating.

By adopting mindful eating choices, improving your awareness, and listening to your body, weight reduction should come naturally and quickly.

26. Focus on Changing Your Lifestyle
Dieting is one of those things that virtually always fails in the long run. Persons who "diet" tend to acquire more weight over time.

Instead of concentrating just on reducing weight, make it a key objective to replenish your body with good food and nutrients.

Eat to become a healthier, happier, fitter person – not only to reduce weight

27. Chew Thoroughly and Slow Down

Your brain needs time to register that you've eaten enough to eat.

Chewing your food fully helps you eat more slowly, which is related to lower food intake, enhanced fullness, and smaller portion sizes.

How soon you complete your meals may also affect your weight.

A recent assessment of 23 observational studies found that quicker eaters are more likely to acquire weight than slower eaters.

Fast eaters are also considerably more prone to be fat.

To get into the habit of eating more slowly, it may help to count how many times you chew each meal.

28. Eat Plenty of Protein

Protein has a profound influence on appetite. It may boost feelings of fullness, decrease appetite and help you consume fewer calories.

This may be because protein affects numerous hormones that play a role in hunger and fullness, including ghrelin and GLP-1.

One research revealed that increasing protein consumption from 15% to 30% of calories helped individuals consume 441 fewer calories per day and lose 11 pounds over 12 weeks, on average, without purposefully limiting any meals.

If you presently have a grain-based breakfast, you may want to consider moving to a protein-rich meal, such as eggs.

In one research, overweight or obese women who had eggs at breakfast ate fewer calories at lunch.